Nutritional Prevention and Cures for Better Health

Natural Alternatives to Restore Your Health

Kelly Larson

Copyright Act of 1976, the scanning, uploading and electronic sharing of any part of this book without the explicit written consent or permission of the publisher constitutes unlawful piracy and the theft of intellectual property.

If you would like to use material or content from this book (other than for review purposes), prior written permission must be obtained from the publisher.

You can contact the publishing company at admin@speedypublishing.com. Thank you for not infringing on the author's rights.

Speedy Publishing LLC (c) 2014
40 E. Main St., #1156
Newark, DE 19711
www.speedypublishing.co

Ordering Information:
Quantity sales; Special discounts are available on quantity purchases by corporations, associations, and others. For details, contact the "Special Sales Department" at the address above.

This is a reprint book.

Manufactured in the United States of America

Table of Contents

Publisher's Notes i

Chapter 1: Health Management Should be Preventative vs. Reactive 1

Chapter 2: How to Boost Your Health to Optimal Levels with Natural Methods 5

Chapter 3: Food Choices Can Prevent or Causing Disease 12

Chapter 4: Eating Well Can Prevent Disease 15

Chapter 5: Control Stress with Good Nutritional Choices 19

Chapter 6: Energy-Boosting Foods that Fight Fatigue 22

Chapter 7: Managing Diabetes with Nutrition 24

Chapter 8: Prevent and Reverse Heart Disease with Proper Nutrition 30

Chapter 9: Non-Inflammatory Foods that Fights Inflammation 36

Chapter 10: Boost Your Memory Function with Nutrition 42

Chapter 11: How to Control and Cure Cancer with Nutrition 48

Meet the Author 54

More Books by Kelly Larson 55

Publisher's Notes

Disclaimer

This publication is intended to provide helpful and informative material. It is not intended to diagnose, treat, cure, or prevent any health problem or condition, nor is intended to replace the advice of a physician. No action should be taken solely on the contents of this book. Always consult your physician or qualified health-care professional on any matters regarding your health and before adopting any suggestions in this book or drawing inferences from it.

The author and publisher specifically disclaim all responsibility for any liability, loss or risk, personal or otherwise, which is incurred as a consequence, directly or indirectly, from the use or application of any contents of this book.

Any and all product names referenced within this book are the trademarks of their respective owners. None of these owners have sponsored, authorized, endorsed, or approved this book.

Always read all information provided by the manufacturers' product labels before using their products. The author and publisher are not responsible for claims made by manufacturers.

Print Edition 2014

Chapter 1: Health Management Should be Preventative vs. Reactive

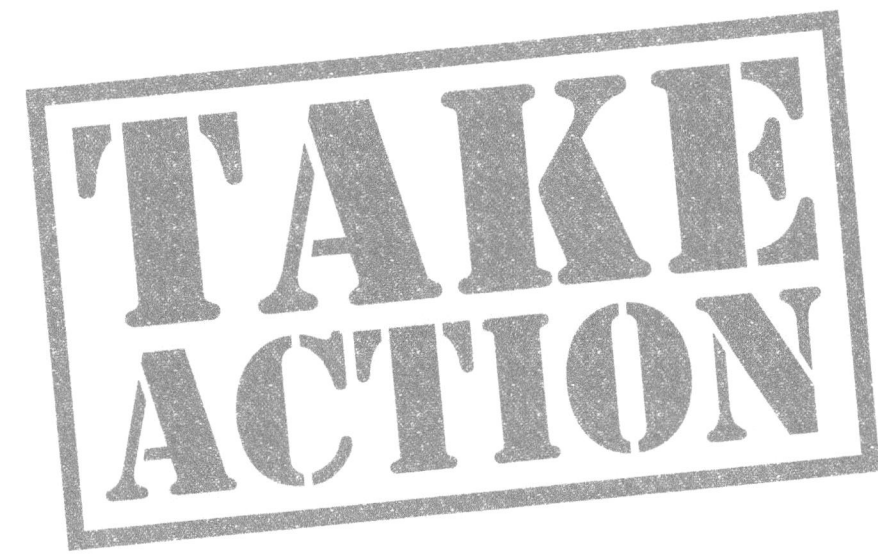

We live in a society where treatment rules over prevention, where the medical community shuns (or hides) natural treatments, and where consumers have to take matters into their own hands if they want to be educated about all of their options.

When it comes to your health, you need to know that you're not at the mercy of your genetics and you don't have to rely on drug treatments for everything.

You also can't rest on your laurels until something bad happens – you need to take a preventative approach to your health while addressing any issues that have already crept up.

Doctors Rarely Discuss Preventative Medicine in Depth

Very few doctors sit down with their patients and help them work out a regimen of preventative medicine.

There's no money in healthy patients, so it's in their best interest – as well as the pharmaceutical companies – to treat you *after* you've already acquired a disease.

It's not all a conspiracy, though. There's not enough time to sit down with a patient and go over a customized plan – not when you're looking at a waiting room full of ill patients.

You, as a consumer, have to take control and educate yourself. You can certainly ask your doctor about his or her recommendations for disease prevention, but you're likely to just get very broad, generic answers – and no details to back it up.

Reliance on prescriptions has become commonplace – so much so that the CDC (Centers for Disease Control), is now issuing warnings about overuse of antibiotics, for example.

Instead of a doctor sitting you down and teaching you how to keep your immune system beefed up so that you won't get sick, for example, he or she simply waits.

When you've come down with something, they then whip out their Rx pad to write you a prescription for antibiotics and steroids and perhaps some cough medicine to quell the symptoms.

You Have Options

There are definitely natural ways to treat things like this – to quell a cough, for example – but you won't hear that from the doctor (or the pharmacist), because that's not where the money is.

Imagine if you knew how to treat the flu on your own. Your doctor wouldn't be able to keep his practice open if everyone were armed with that information! So you're kept in the dark.

Prescriptions are expensive – whether you're paying for them out of pocket or your insurance company is paying for them. Eventually, it comes out of your pocket through increased premiums.

There are many ways to treat and prevent disease.

Food is one source. Healing your body (or strengthening it) from the inside out, helps you develop cells that can battle disease before they take root in your body.

There are also alternative and holistic measures you can take to create your own treatment and healing plan. You might want a combination of natural and traditional disease prevention.

For example, you get your kids immunized against disease to help protect them. But you also teach them how to wash their hands to prevent the spread of germs – and you feed them immune-boosting foods that help keep them healthy and fend of attacks by germs.

You can do the same with disease. When it comes to cancer, for example – you want to eat plenty of antioxidants, but you also want to have cancer screenings to catch any disease that occurs.

If you do develop the disease, you'll probably embark on a journey to get the very best medical treatment available to you in the traditional sense. But you also will probably find information about nutrition and other treatments that help heal cancer naturally.

Chapter 2: How to Boost Your Health to Optimal Levels with Natural Methods

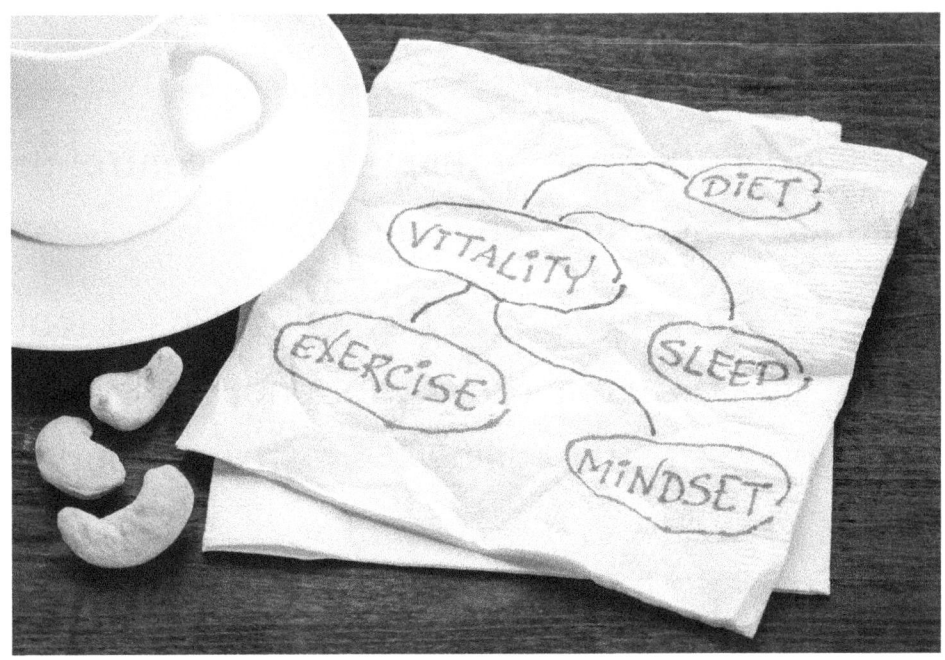

In order to better manage your health, you need to take a five-point approach to preventing and healing your body. We're going to go over all five right now, but then pick the most important one to focus on in depth – nutrition.

Sleep

Getting enough rest is imperative in allowing your body to do its work to repair your body at a cellular level. Many people suffer from sleep issues – some slightly and some who suffer from extreme insomnia.

It's a proven fact that those who don't get enough sleep often endure consequences for it – like increased risk of diabetes, high blood pressure and coronary disease.

This is only part of the problem. These same individuals are often plagued with stress because they're not getting enough sleep, so they end up spiraling down into a deep depression.

When these factors combine, it leads to a shortened life expectancy. Luckily, this is something you can control naturally – it doesn't require dangerous sleeping pills.

Start with better sleep hygiene. Take a good, hard look at how your sleep set-up is. Is your room cool enough? Is it quiet and dark? Are your sheets, pillows, mattress and blankets comfortable?

What do you do before bed? It shouldn't be stimulating to your mind. Read; take a bath – but stay off the electronic gadgets. If you've done all of that and still aren't sleeping, then you can use nutrition to help you get more sleep!

Foods rich in antioxidants help you get more sleep. Make sure the foods are packed with vitamin C and selenium. This is perfect for those who don't get enough sleep – but what about those who sleep, and still feel tired anyway?

Sometimes quality of sleep is what makes the difference. Try eating an ounce of dark chocolate and adding some turkey and eggs to your nutritional regimen. This will help send you into that deep, relaxing slumber you need to awaken feeling refreshed.

Exercise

Moving your body is a great, natural way to stave off disease and reverse health problems you may have. Researchers know that it has the ability to prevent and heal heart disease.

It also helps reverse diabetes – and many people find that they're able to get off of insulin because of their combined nutrition and exercise plan. Hopping on a treadmill and getting some cardio into your day can benefit you if you have high blood pressure, too.

As for prevention, those who exercise have a smaller risk of developing colon cancer. And if osteoporosis is a concern, then moving your body will help strengthen, not weaken, your bones.

You want to engage in exercise that gives your whole body a workout. When you engage in cardiovascular exercise, like jogging or aerobics, then your heart gains strength, your blood pressure is kept under control, and your cholesterol levels benefit.

Believe it or not, nutrition factors in heavily to your workout success. Your body uses food as fuel to get you through all of your workouts – and it helps you recover from them, too.

Carbs are very important for people doing high levels of activity. And it's the amino acids in protein that assist you in repairing the muscles that you break down when you're strength-training.

Nutrition

We'll get into this in much more detail shortly, but let's touch on how important food is to your well-being. Growing up, you probably heard little snippets of advice – like how chicken broth helps cure a cold.

And it's not an old wives' tale, either! Researchers at the University of Nebraska Medical Center in Omaha broke it down and discovered that the properties found in chicken broth really do suppress the symptoms of a common cold.

There are many ways that food can help your body. You've already seen some of the healing properties being discussed, like protein being necessary for your muscles to heal after a workout.

You can also boost your immune system, increase your memory retention, and keep many major diseases (heart disease, diabetes, cancer, etc.) at bay – just by using food to empower your body at a cellular level.

Stress Relief

Stress is one of the primary issues men and women (and even teens) suffer from today that result in poor health. In fact, it's estimated that 70-90% of all doctor's visits originate from stress.

Stress starts off as a reaction in your body that you see as mental. It's your mind's reaction to something that angers or saddens you. But your body is undergoing a physical reaction beneath the surface.

It's flooded with cortisol, the "fight or flight" hormone. This isn't harmful on occasion, but if you suffer from chronic daily stress, it starts to take a toll on your body, and you will begin seeing increased symptoms of disease.

For example, stress directly affects your insulin levels. It has the ability to keep your blood pressure raised to dangerous levels. It also hinders your chance to steer clear of (or recover from) cancer.

The National Cancer Institute reports that there's evidence that stress affects your clinical results for becoming cancer-free with treatment. Stress causes common health issues, too, including:

- Flu
- Insomnia
- Digestive issues
- Urinary problems
- Infertility
- Headaches

You have to get it under control *before* you turn to a doctor for help with his or her prescription pad. What's the best way to do that? You can have your pick of many options.

You can use exercise to release endorphins, food to deliver a calming state of mind, mind relaxation techniques such as neuro-linguistic programming, emotional freedom technique, or even meditation. If you just need a little help, you might turn to aromatherapy or massage for the stress relief you need.

Elimination of Risky Behaviors

One of the best things you can do for your health is to get rid of the risks that you're taking. Increasing healthy behaviors (like stress relief, nutrition, sleep and exercise) are just part of the equation.

What can you eliminate?

Drinking is always touted in medical articles as having the ability to benefit you. While it's true that some moderate alcohol has been shown to benefit heart health, overuse only contributes to the probability of disease.

Smoking is never good – regardless of what they told people in the old days. We now know how harmful it is to you – and to those around you. Not only are you upping your chances of developing lung disease, but because it constricts your blood flow, you'll be setting yourself up for heart disease, too.

Doing drugs – prescription or otherwise – will eventually take a toll on your body. Your cells can't recover quickly from a drug-induced state, so your entire body becomes weakened against infection and disease.

Risky sexual behaviors are also common. While you might think something like herpes simplex is just a mere nuisance, it actually increases your risk of acquiring major diseases like HIV if you're not careful about keeping outbreaks under control and your immune system high.

As you can see, you have a whole host of options available to you to help prevent and reverse disease. Unfortunately, most of us don't live a healthy lifestyle – we just run to the doctor once something bad happens.

If you're tired of living like this, and ready to become more reliant on yourself than you are a prescription pad, then it's time you find a good starting point to manage your health.

Nutrition is the most powerful weapon you have against disease – and it's something you have to engage in daily anyway. Nobody's going to ask you to give up your favorite foods forever.

The key is to add nutrients and optimize your menu wherever possible so that your cells have a chance to flourish and the unhealthy toxins in your body are flushed out so they can't continue to do more damage.

Chapter 3: Food Choices Can Prevent or Causing Disease

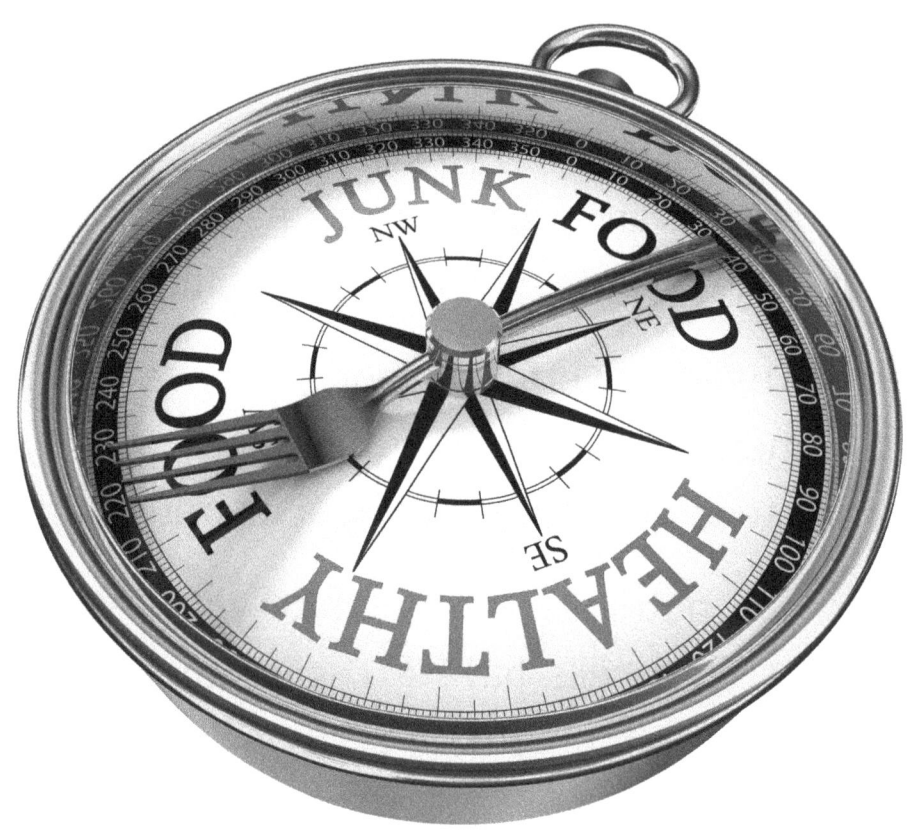

For many people, disease isn't something that's considered until they actually head to the doctor and get a diagnosis. Sometimes, if a disease runs in the family, it's given more consideration, but most people don't take a preventative approach to their health care.

Imagine if you could actually *see* disease forming within your body. What if you knew when every single cell turned cancerous – or every time your arteries accumulated a little more plaque build-up?

It would be alarming, for sure. But we don't see it. Some of us prefer to not think about it, but if you want to live a long and healthy life, it's time you started imagining what's happening with every bite of food you consume.

That cupcake you just ate? It sent your blood sugar levels spiraling out of control. Your arteries wound up just a teeny bit thicker because of the fat it was made with.

The cancer cells in your body love the increased sugar because it's what they thrive on. Your memories will suffer just a bit. And if you're prone to inflammation, then this type of food choice will ensure a nice flare-up for you shortly.

Think of another food that might be a better option. For example, if you had grabbed a handful of walnuts instead. Walnuts are packed with vitamin E, which offers protection for your heart.

Cancer cells, blood sugar and inflammation are no match for the elements found in walnuts. It's known as a super food because it has powerful benefits. If you're worried about diabetes or cancer, this is a food you should be consuming daily.

Food often helps or hurt you in terms of disease. Cooking meat, for example can lead to increased cancer risk (if you char your food) – or increased heart protection (if you ate broiled salmon).

Every time you sit down to eat, look at your plate and figure out if what you're about to eat – and the way it's prepared – is going to do harm to your body, or help it thrive at a cellular level that you can't see with the naked eye.

Sometimes you can make better choices, like baking or broiling instead of frying – or going organic instead of eating foods covered in pesticides. You're the only person who can steer your health in the right direction, but it forces you to become thoughtful about your choices.

Chapter 4: Eating Well Can Prevent Disease

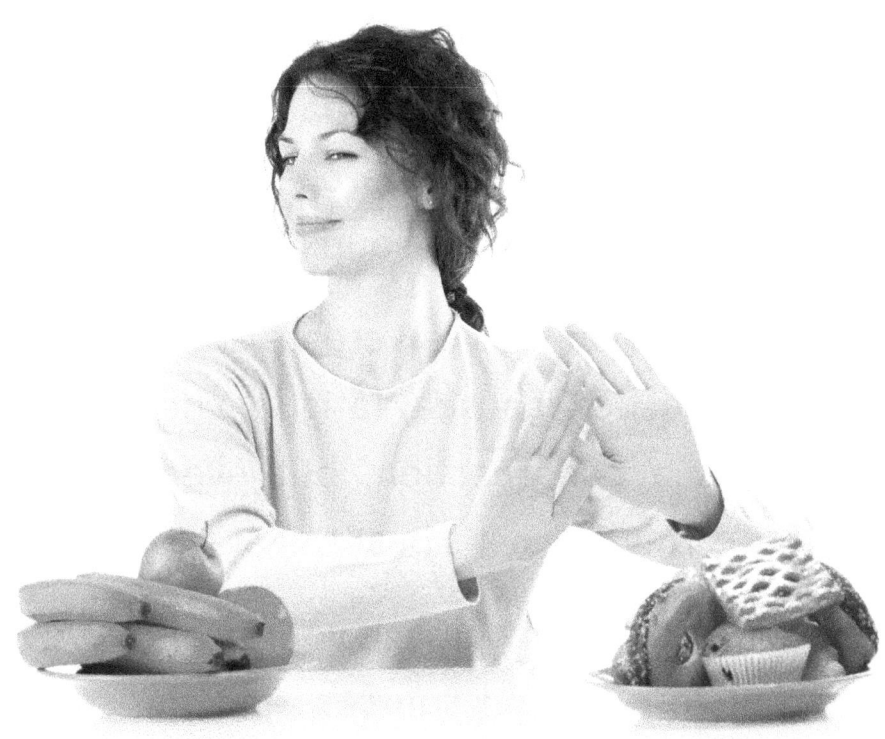

When you're ready to adopt a lifestyle change where you're using food to fuel and heal your body instead of for comfort, it means you have to look at what's going in, what needs to be eliminated, and what you can add for better health.

There are two steps to this process. First, get rid of the foods that are damaging our body from a cellular level. Second, start feeding yourself foods that help boost your body's ability to survive and thrive.

Weeding Out Foods That Are Toxic to Your Body

We live in a culture where ingredients are added into our meals and processed foods in a way where we're rarely, if ever, aware of them. Sometimes we've just been raised to turn to certain foods for comfort, so we don't view a doughnut (for example) as a toxin, but as something that brings us pleasure.

MSG is known as monosodium glutamate. You regularly find it in Chinese food, but it's also found in processed meats that you eat, as well as some canned foods like soups and vegetables.

This is an additive to food that can create a toxic reaction in your body, such as headaches, nausea, fatigue, chest pain and more. Not everyone has a bad reaction, but even if you feel mild discomfort after eating MSG, it's best to get rid of it in your diet.

Salt is an ingredient that can damage your health. We're routinely adding extra salt to our food sources, and this isn't necessary. Almost all foods (even sweet ones) have salt in them.

The guidelines say that if you're fifty or under, you should limit your salt intake to 2,300 milligrams per day. If you're older than fifty, you should slash it almost in half – to 1,500 milligrams per day.

You should never stop using salt completely – because you'll suffer from negative side effects just as you do when you're consuming too much salt. You need just the right balance.

Sugar isn't just found in sweets. It's hidden in many seemingly healthy foods, such as low-fat and light foods. Even some foods labeled whole grain are packed with grams of sugar – so you have to be vigilant about what you consume.

It's been reported that Americans typically eat three pounds of sugar per person *per week*. How does it affect your health? Not only does it damage your immune system, but it also feeds cancer cells, contributes to obesity (and diabetes), and boosts your risk for heart disease.

Gluten is one ingredient that many people have a negative health reaction to. While many health plans tout grains as a main staple of your meal plans, gluten is found in grains – and it can cause you to have allergic reactions that complicate your health.

Embrace a Basic Health-Driven Nutritional Plan

Unless you're already suffering from a major medical disease, then you should strive for a healthy, Mediterranean-style diet. This type of diet feeds your body the foods it needs to protect your organs and overall health.

It's based on a heart-healthy idea, but if you're following this type of nutritional regimen, you'll be helping other parts of your body as well. A Mediterranean diet consists of:

- Fruits
- Vegetables
- Whole Grains
- Nuts
- Olive Oil
- Seeds

- Legumes
- Beans
- Herbs and Spices

You should eat healthy fish a couple of times a week, dairy and poultry periodically, and red meat and sugary foods infrequently. While whole grains are a main part of this eating style, that doesn't mean you have to eat gluten-heavy grains. You can eat gluten-free grains like corn, quinoa, wild rice, millet, and buckwheat.

Sometimes disease has already hit your life. Next, let's look at five common health issues and how your nutrition plan can assist you in treating or curing them.

Chapter 5: Control Stress with Good Nutritional Choices

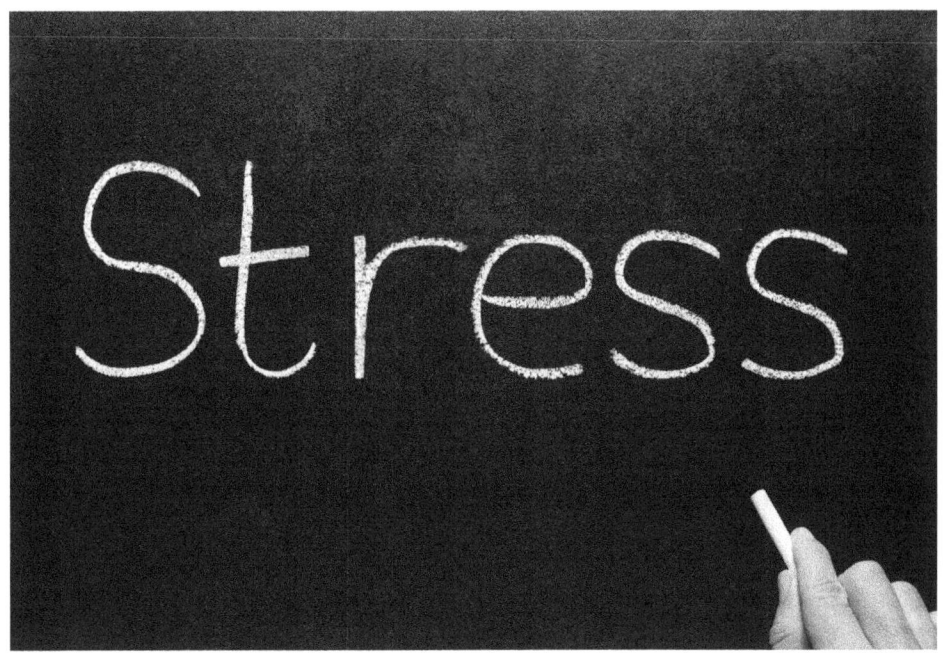

When someone mentions the words "food" and "stress" in the same sentence, you're probably instantly looking at the connection between too much stresses and using food as comfort.

There's nothing wrong with enjoying food. We've always been a society where meals are meant for bonding with friends and family. Of course, using it in an unhealthy way, to suppress feelings, is never good.

But did you know there's another way to look at the food and stress connection? Certain foods can actually *help* you in the stress relief department – you just have to know which foods to choose over cakes and other unhealthy carbs.

There are foods that suppress cortisol in your body. Cortisol is the hormone that is released in your body when you're under stress. It makes you feel that "fight or flight" feeling.

It's not bad once in a while, but chronic cortisol can damage your body at a cellular level. Instead, you want foods that keep cortisol under control, like nuts, for instance! It doesn't take many, but a handful of nuts allow the magnesium to keep cortisol levels in balance.

Do you think your blood pressure spikes when you're stressed out? It probably does. If this is a danger to you, or you want to feel calmer, reach for a food high in potassium like a banana or an avocado.

Asparagus, which is rich in folic acid, helps boost your mood, which directly combats that stressed-out feeling. Broccoli does the same thing. Eat it raw so that the nutrients don't get zapped through the cooking process.

Sugary foods combat stress, too. Didn't expect to hear that, did you? But all it takes is a teeny amount on your tongue to do the job, so eat a fruit-filled sorbet with natural sugars instead of full fat ice cream.

Stress takes a toll on your body. With cortisol coursing through your veins, your cells have a hard time repairing what goes wrong. That's why your immune system takes a hit when you're stressed. Foods rich in antioxidants and vitamin C, like blueberries, can help you feel calm and healthier during stressful times.

Are you the type of person who goes on full alert when you're stressed out? If your adrenaline gets pumping, opt for an oily, omega-3 filled fish to help soothe your mood.

We mentioned cakes and fatty carbs initially. Carbs can actually help keep you calm by boosting serotonin levels, but choose whole grain options instead. Complex carbs don't have you crashing like the others do.

CHAPTER 6: ENERGY-BOOSTING FOODS THAT FIGHT FATIGUE

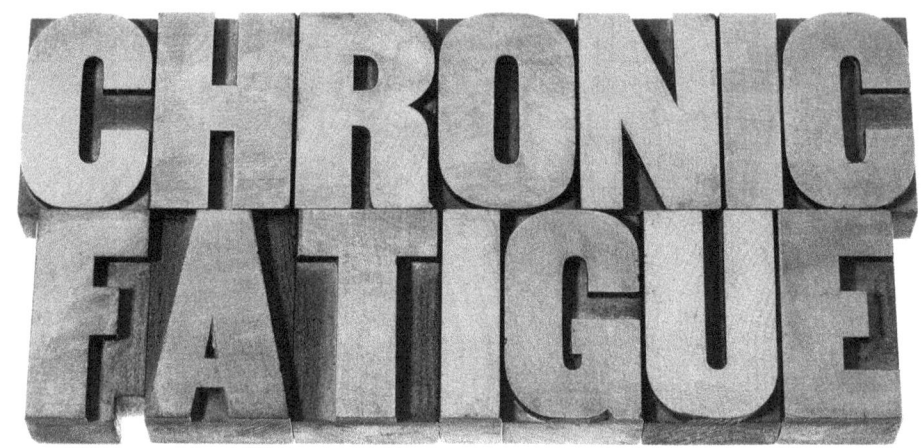

Feeling sluggish every day? You're not alone. Many men and women wake up tired, and go through their day feeling exhausted. In an effort to stay awake and function, they turn to food – but it's the sugary, high caffeine options that have them crashing thirty minutes to an hour later.

You *can* use food to provide energy to your body, but it has to be done the right way. For instance, if you're used to eating a chocolate candy bar for energy, then switch to a couple of ounces of dark chocolate instead.

You get the caffeine and sugar, but also the health benefits of this wonderful food and in moderation, you won't suffer from the typical sugar crash you have after a milk chocolate candy bar.

Flavor your meal with some spicy herbs for a quick energy boost. Foods with capsaicin – like hot chili peppers – can boost your energy and provide other health benefits, too.

If you need a snack to wake up and get tasks done, reach for a banana. The potassium helps keep your blood sugar levels stable so that you don't have that midday crash in energy.

A great high fiber, high carb snack that won't pack on pounds is popcorn. Eat the healthier versions, not those laden with tons of movie theater butter slathered all over it.

Iron-rich foods like leafy green vegetables can supply you with tons of energy. When your iron levels wane, it makes you feel weak and lethargic. Try greens like kale, spinach, collard, mustards and turnips.

Fresh fruit can do the job! Grab a handful of grapes, or use citrus fruits as a quick pick-me-up. Oranges, or even lemon added to your water, can perk you up if you start slumping.

Find a food cooked with curry! Not only is it delicious, but curry stabilized blood sugar to prevent crashes – and it also helps with the circulation in your body to keep your body well oxygenated.

And don't forget water. Although it's a drink and not a food, it's what helps keep your body operating in tip top shape at a cellular level. Without proper hydration, it won't matter what foods you eat because the nutrients won't be able to do their job.

Chapter 7: Managing Diabetes with Nutrition

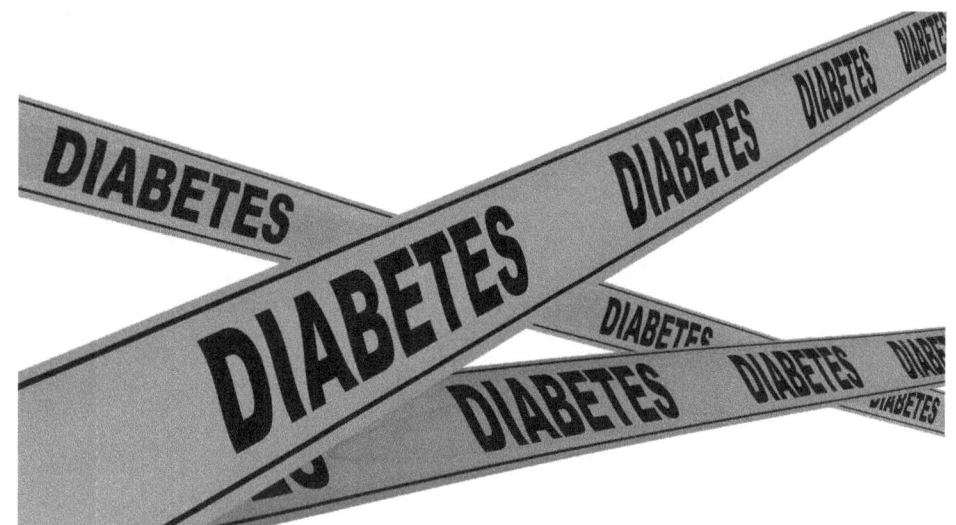

There's a big misconception when it comes to diabetes nutrition. Some people mistakenly think that all you have to do is cut out sugar forever and you'll be just fine.

That's not true.

You have to eat strategically in order to keep your blood glucose levels in order. If you're diabetic, it also means you have to plan *when* you eat – not just *what* you eat.

If you skip meals, it can make your diabetes worse – and yet, eating in moderation and losing weight can reverse diabetes so that you're no longer dependent on insulin.

It's important to keep your blood sugar levels at a range of 70-130 milligrams per deciliter on a regular basis. It should spike to no more than 180 mg/dL a couple of hours after you eat.

What Not to Eat as a Diabetic

The worst thing you can do is deprive yourself of your favorite foods so that you end up binging on them and causing your insulin levels to spike to dangerous levels.

However, you should also make better food choices whenever possible. When it comes to sweets, for example, there are diabetic-friendly options. Fried chips aren't good for you, but baked chips are better.

Following our plan of ridding your body of toxic foods first, let's look at the worst foods you can eat if you're a diabetic. You want to adhere to a meal plan made up of mostly foods that are low on the Glycemic Index.

That means these foods spike your insulin levels the least amount. You can find foods ranked on this index so that you know what kinds of changes it will cause in your body.

Foods that are bad for your blood glucose include:

- White bread
- Pasta
- White potatoes
- Popcorn
- Candy
- Cereal
- Watermelon
- Pineapple

If you do add a food high on the glycemic index, then you can balance it out with foods lower on the scale, too. Try to moderate the portions that you consume – and watch out for seemingly healthy foods (like raisins), which have an unhealthy volume of natural sugars in them.

While you're managing your meals, fueling your body throughout the day with foods that aren't detrimental to your health, you want to also lay off the sodas – including diet drinks.

Drink plenty of water instead. Even juice, which sounds healthy because it comes from a fruit, is often packed with sugar that can harm your recovery plans as a diabetic.

Feed Your Body the Right Food for Diabetes

After ridding yourself of toxins that keep your body in a perpetual state of insulin dependency, you'll want to begin reversing this health problem by feeding your body foods that help it maintain balance.

There are certain foods that are superb for diabetics to eat.

Start by trying to add dark, leafy green vegetables into your meal plan. From spinach with your omelet to a side of greens at lunch and dinner, this super food helps diabetics feel full without overloading them on unhealthy carbs and too many calories.

Kale is one of the best leafy greens to eat. But there are others (in addition to spinach), too. You can try a variety to see what taste you prefer – such as mustard green, collard greens, and turnip greens.

While pizza might not be healthy for a diabetic, the tomato sauce *is*. Pasta isn't usually a good option, so what you can do is get your supply of tomatoes either by eating them raw or in a sauce poured over whole grain pasts instead.

Tomatoes are healthy for diabetics because they're full of vitamins and nutrients. They include vitamin E and C as well as plenty of iron. You can get tomatoes in the form of soup, too – but make sure that however you eat them, you're checking to see how much added sugar is in the product and how many carbs it's loaded with.

Beans are a great food for diabetics. The fiber they pack is virtually unparalleled. They're also very filing, and you get a lot of potassium and magnesium in each serving.

Even though they're starches, they're packed with protein, so you can forego the saturated fat that's found in meat and eat healthy beans instead. The soluble fiber in beans binds to the carbs and helps slow the digestive process, keeping your insulin levels stable.

Potatoes are a food that aren't usually good for diabetics, but those are Russet potatoes – not the sweet potatoes, which are one of the diabetic super foods you can eat.

White potatoes have a high GI but sweet potatoes have a low GI, and they're full of fiber and vitamin A. You can bake them whole or cut them into fries and bake them for a healthy snack.

If you're diabetic, following a Mediterranean diet can be beneficial for you – especially if you eat fish that's high in Omega-3 fatty acids. That includes salmon and tuna – but make sure it's cooked in a healthy manner, like baked or broiled.

When it comes to fruit, not all fruit is good for a diabetic person to eat. But some can help – such as citrus options – oranges, grapefruit, and even lemons and limes – which you can put in your water for a flavorful option. You get fiber and vitamin C – and it helps boost your immune system in the process.

Bread is a hard thing to give up, but white bread is something that can cause a spike in your blood glucose. Go with whole grain options instead. That way you get some omega-3 fatty acids, folate and chromium to help your body heal, too.

Some of the other foods that are perfect for diabetics include berries (all kinds) – for their fiber and nutrients as well as nuts and seeds, such as walnuts and flax seeds, which fill you with fiber and help, stave off hunger for long periods of time.

Dairy products can be tricky. Just make sure you choose healthy diary that's not flooded with sugar. You need the vitamin D for strong bones and healthy teeth, but you don't want the spike in insulin.

When it comes to shopping for foods to treat and reverse diabetes, stick to the outer edge of the grocery store, away from the processed foods that won't serve your body well.

Chapter 8: Prevent and Reverse Heart Disease with Proper Nutrition

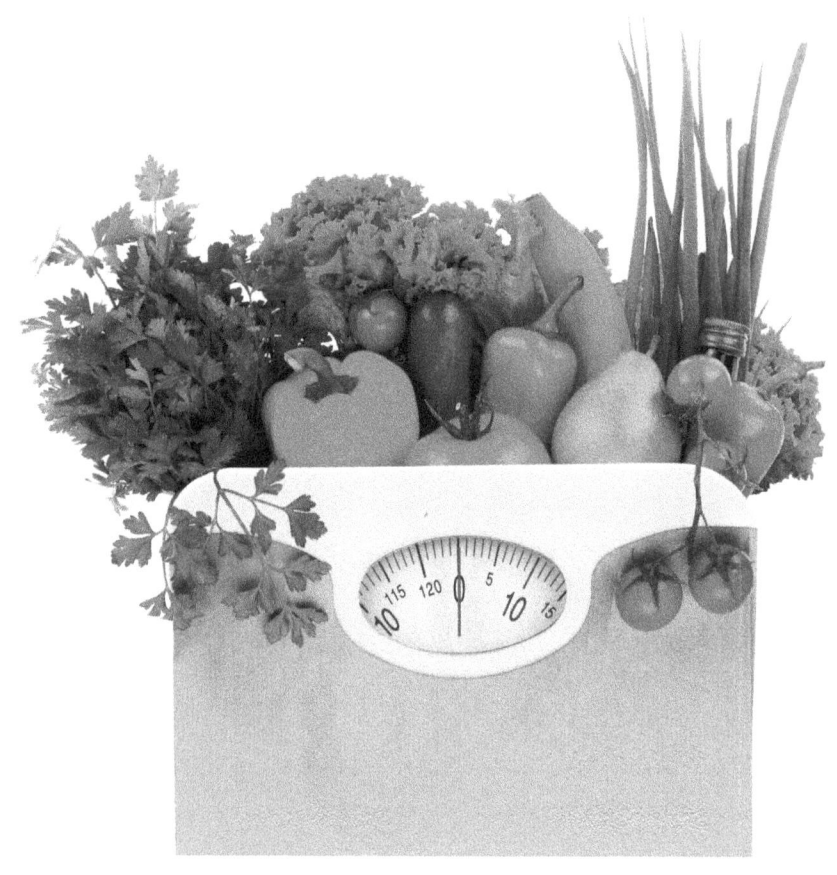

Heart disease is a health issue that sneaks up on you. You typically don't know that you're suffering from it until you begin experiencing dangerous symptoms. Regardless of whether you've already confirmed that you have heart disease, or you're trying to ensure you never get it, you can use food to manage the situation to a large degree.

Heart disease is when your arteries are becoming partially or fully blocked from the build-up of plaque, cutting off the blood supply to your heart and causing portions of it to die.

Heart disease is the number one killer of both men and women in the United States, so you definitely want to adhere to a diet that helps break up plaque in your arteries even if you're not showing signs of the disease just yet.

Eliminate Plaque Building Foods from Your Diet

The first thing you want to do is be kind to your body in terms of portion sizes. While it can handle a little bit of the "bad" foods, your body can become overwhelmed when you're eating enough for three people.

If you're used to consuming huge portions, it can be tough to suddenly cut back – so choose low calorie, healthy foods like dark, leafy greens that you can basically eat an unlimited amount of.

In our steps to use nutrition to fight back against disease, you first want to look at what you need to eat less (if any) of. That includes trans-fat, like the kinds found in fried foods (think doughnuts).

Red meat and whole fat dairy has a lot of trans-fat, too – but you can choose better options, like lean meats (not marbled) and low-fat milk options such as 1% or skim.

Watch out for other dairy foods like cheese and ice cream. Some of them are high in fat and will clog your arteries quickly, as will any highly processed meats, such as hot dogs and sandwich meat.

Whenever you go to the store, try buying as many fresh ingredients as possible. Prepackaged foods are usually high in sodium (salt), and this contributes to heart disease, too – so stay away from those.

We'll talk about which fruits and vegetables to fuel your body with shortly, but there are also some you want to avoid. It's great to eat vegetables and fruits, but don't buy prepackages vegetables slathered in cream-based sauces, or fruit canned with a high sugar syrup.

Grains are a staple of a heart-healthy diet, but not grains that have been processed and stripped of their nutrients. Avoid white grains, like white bread, cakes, biscuits, and even some seemingly healthy muffins.

When you're cooking, you want to stay away from fats that are solid at room temperature, like butter or margarine. Instead, use healthier fats like olive oil, which help reverse signs of heart disease.

Some people think that if a product has "coconut oil" listed as an ingredient, then it must be healthy. But coconut oil isn't friendly to your heart health, so look for that as an ingredient and steer clear.

You always want to stick to a diet that will keep your LDL (bad) cholesterol levels low and your HDL (good) cholesterol levels high. A study was performed by the Harvard School of Public

Health, which surveyed Americans and found out that the most common and most harmful plaque-building foods we eat are:

- Cheese
- Pizza
- Desserts made of grains (like cakes)
- Desserts made of dairy (like ice cream)
- Chicken
- Pork
- Beef
- Milk
- Pasta
- Eggs
- Candy
- Butter

Of course, when you look at the above list, you can probably instantly spot some immediate healthier substitutes you can make just by choosing low fat options or whole grain options instead of full fat or white, processed ones.

Add in Foods That Clear Plaque and Boost Heart Health

Some foods will harm your heart health depending on how you cook them. For instance, chicken can be prepared healthfully, but if you leave the skin on and fry it, it won't be healthy at all.

If you've prepared a meal from scratch, such as a soup or stew, and you're reheating it as a leftover meal. Try to skim the solidified fat off the top and throw it away before you turn on the stove.

Your heart needs a good balance of lean meats, fruits, vegetables, whole grains, nuts and seeds. You're looking for lots of fiber to help flush out the plaque from your system.

Some of the best grains to eat include:

- Whole grain bread and pasta
- High fiber cereal and oatmeal
- Brown rice
- Flaxseed

Vegetables should be a staple in your diet. Asparagus and bell peppers (which have tons of B6) help keep your homocysteine levels low – something that contributes to heart disease. Try to get a rainbow of vegetables in your diet. Combined with fruits, you should be aiming for eight or more servings per day. Choose fresh, not canned or frozen options.

Nuts like almonds and walnuts – as well as seeds – all have a heart healthy effect on your body. These are filling snacks – you can grab a handful of almonds instead of a dessert cake and feel full for hours.

Meat should be as healthy as you can find it. Salmon and tuna are best for their Omega-3 benefits, but if you go with red meat, choose lean, un-marbled varieties.

Managing your heart health can be as simple as making small tweaks to your diet, or it might requires you to do a full overhaul of your nutrition plan. Keep in mind that exercise can help protect your heart, too!

Chapter 9: Non-Inflammatory Foods that Fights Inflammation

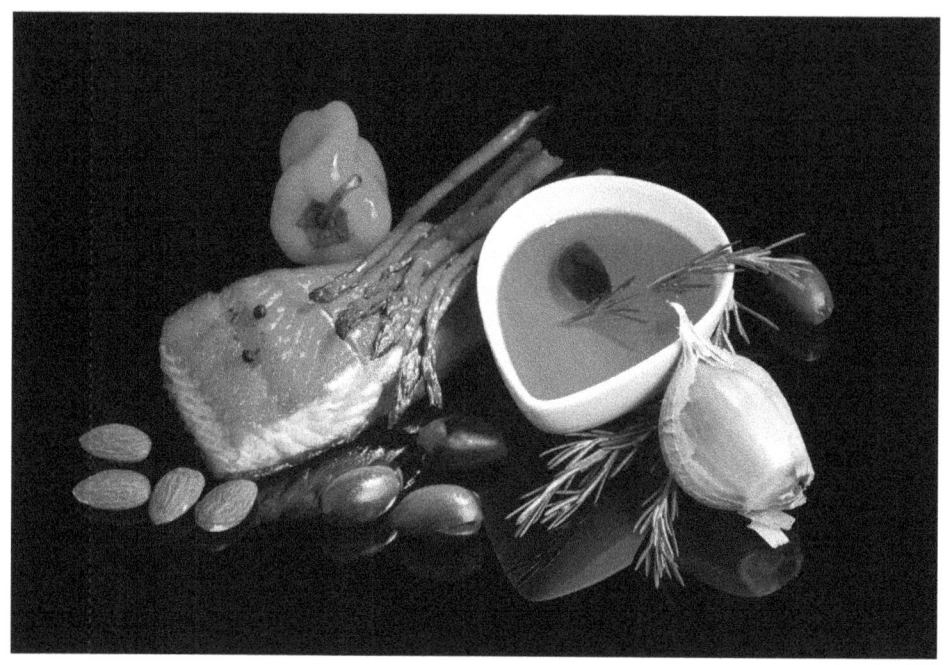

While inflammation isn't necessarily anything that will cut your longevity short, it *is* something that quickly deteriorates your quality of life. Living in pain isn't something anyone wants to experience.

Inflammation is when your body is trying to protect you, but it ends up creating pain instead. It hones in on something that needs to be attacked – like irritants or unhealthy cells – and normally, it would help heal you.

But inflammation takes a wrong turn when it actually goes too far and the inflammation hurts more than the infection. You can tell if you have inflammation because you'll experience pain, swelling, and redness.

It can benefit you, for instance if you hurt your knee, because it alerts you to the fact that you've damaged your tissues – so it helps you go easy on your joints until the tissue is able to heal.

However, the inflammation sometimes makes it harder to recover, and more inflammation occurs because of the initial flare-up, so you need something to quell the inflammation – and food can be your helper!

Inflammation in and of itself isn't life threatening. But it's been linked to other health concerns like diabetes and cancer. If you go to the doctor for a health concern, you'll find that many diagnoses turn out to have some level of inflammation – such as a swollen throat due to a common cold. So even if it's not terminal, keeping inflammation at bay helps you live a healthier life.

Toxic Foods That Cause Inflammation Flare-Ups

Adhering to our "remove and replace" regimen for fighting disease with foods, there are certain items you want to restrict or rid from your diet as much as possible.

- Alcohol
- Fried foods
- Processed meats (bacon, hot dogs, bologna)
- Eggs
- Coffee

If you have arthritis, then your doctor probably told you to steer clear of these inflammation-worsening foods. It's typically beneficial for you to stick to a Mediterranean type diet – one where meat is limited and fruits, whole grains and vegetables are paramount.

Freshness counts, too. Eating all of those high sugar, high salt processed foods that come prepackaged worsen your inflammation and cause more pain in your body.

If you can, switch to a mostly vegetarian diet. Meats tend to flare up inflammation, so if you have to eat meat, make them a small portion on your plate and not a main attraction.

The saturated fats found in animal protein actually help create inflammation because it contains arachidonic acid. U.S. News reported that diets that don't have as much of this molecule have a lower incidence of inflammation flare-ups.

Dairy can be inflammatory to your body, too. Things like full fat butter, cheese, milk and yogurt do nothing good for your body If you eat dairy products, choose low-fat or skim versions.

Sweeteners – real and artificial – can cause inflammation in your body. Everything from fried or baked cakes to soft drinks can worsen your symptoms of pain and swelling.

Wheat and gluten products can lead to increased inflammation in your body. You want to look for gluten-free foods as much as possible to keep the reaction out of your body.

Many people who suffer from inflammation conditions know the effect that alcohol has on them. It unfortunately contains a high amount of sugar, which contributes to a raised level of inflammation.

Heal Your Body through Non-Inflammatory Foods

So what *should* you eat to control and reverse symptoms of inflammation in your body? The key is to keep your system from attacking itself, so that means boosting the health of your body at a cellular level.

Food can help with this.

Again, the Mediterranean diet is the perfect recipe for success when it comes to keeping inflammation at bay. Instead of marbled meat, choose Omega-3 packed fish, like salmon or tuna a few times a week.

Soy is a great meat alternative. This estrogen-like plant-based food helps lower inflammation in your body. But it all depends on how processed it is. Try for more natural versions like tofu and edamame.

Eating foods like spinach, kale, turnip greens, collard greens or mustard greens can have a positive effect on your inflammation issues. They contain tons of vitamin E, which protects your body from cytokines – the molecules that help inflammation occur.

Dairy is something that's good for your bones, but full fat dairy can cause inflammation. Some people have mistakenly thought that they had to stay away from all dairy, but low fat variations are good for you.

If you don't have any allergic reactions to dairy, then look for dairy products that have a double benefit for inflammation – like yogurt with probiotics. This helps inflammation in the gut.

Grains aren't always good for you, but in the case of inflammation, whole grains can help reduce pain and swelling. The fiber in whole grains helps suppress the C-reactive protein, which helps flare-ups.

Nuts are a food that can tame inflammation in your body. Look for nuts like walnuts and almonds, which have tons of fiber, calcium, omega-3 fatty acids and vitamin E. They also have antioxidants to help repair inflammation in your body.

Here's a food that seems like it would cause flare-ups, but which actually heals your body – peppers! You can choose peppers that aren't hot, like bell peppers, or spicy peppers like chili or cayenne peppers.

The one thing that causes heat – the capsaicin, will actually help your pain and swelling go down. Manufacturers even use it in topical creams for arthritis and other inflammation disorders.

Here's what you need to know about inflammation – treatments aren't a one size fits all solution. One person might have an allergic reaction to something and have their inflammation worsen, while another feels healed and whole after trying a particular nutritional solution.

You have to keep track of what works and what doesn't and tailor your anti-inflammatory diet to your own personal preferences and reactions. Eliminate foods that cause flare-ups, and eat more of those that suppress the inflammation in your body.

Chapter 10: Boost Your Memory Function with Nutrition

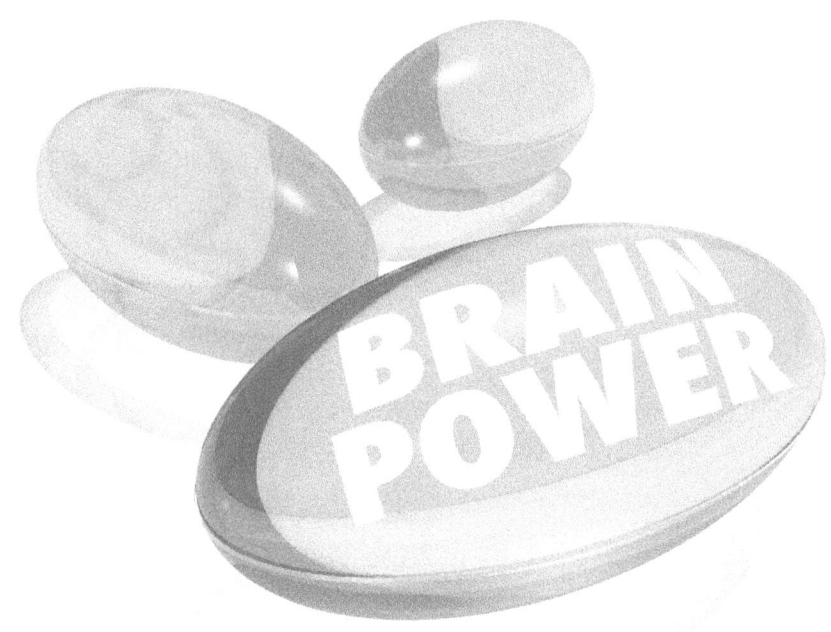

One of the most feared health issues for many men and women is the loss of brain function. Memories, in particular, are treasured and irreplaceable. So it's important that you do everything in your power to protect your mind.

Alzheimer's disease is one memory disease that hits particularly hard, but it's not the only one. Some aging citizens suffer from milder forms of dementia, too. You can protect your mind in many ways.

Some people like to work on their mental clarity and memory retention by exercising it with strategy games and puzzles. Playing Sudoku, for example, can help you with your brain health.

But food can also help (or hurt) your memory function.

Ridding Your Body of Memory-Stealing Toxins

The brain is a very sensitive thing. Deficiencies can cause permanent damage, but so can the flood of toxins in your body that impair your cognitive function. You have to know what harms your brain so that you can replace it with memory boosting foods instead.

One thing scientists are concerned about is that men and women are consuming foods that result in brain plaque. Similar to how arterial plaque can block blood flow and result in coronary disease, it's thought that brain plaque can impair your memory.

Nutritional Neuroscience reported on a study about a protein called amyloid beta, which is a sign of brain plaque. When your brain is able to break down this protein, you don't suffer from memory ailments like you do when the brain is unable to break it down and it hardens and builds up.

Your cells begin to die off instead of strengthening their connections and eventually, you start showing signs of impairment – like walking into a room and forgetting why you are there, or not understanding how to drive home from familiar places.

Sugar is one thing that has the potential to harm your memory capabilities. When we think of sugar intake, we're usually concerned with diabetes and obesity, but it also hurts your brain function.

The Journal of Physiology published a study about how high intake of sugar leads to long term cognitive decline. Things like sugary sodas and cakes were to blame – not naturally occurring sugars like those found in sweet fruit.

In the studies, the lab rats that showed signs of illness from high sugar intake were helped significantly when Omega-3 fatty acids were introduced to their diets.

Some of the foods we focus on in terms of obesity (trans fats like potato chips, solid fats and candy) can do tremendous damage to your mind. Not only have studies shown that memory function decreases for those who eat a diet rich in these substances, but they also show less brain volume, and lower scoring on tests for these individuals.

Processed foods are harmful to your nutritional needs when it comes to repairing or retaining memory function. You want to stick to a diet rich in fresh food sources, not packaged for long-term shelf life.

Get Plenty of These Foods for Increased Brain Function

Whenever your body is low on B12 and iron, your mind doesn't function as sharply – and that includes recalling information of a short or long term nature. Foods that provide plenty of these nutrients can help significantly.

Researchers say that it's crucial to your mind that you preserve the connections of your nerve cells – and antioxidants can help you in that regard. You can get these in various fruits and vegetables that you consumer.

In lab studies, science proved that living beings that consumed plenty of berries, leafy greens and foods packed with vitamin E suffered fewer instances of memory loss than those who didn't.

Mice that were fed a diet of blueberries instead of the usual rat food show significant abilities to break down the amyloid protein that built up in other rodents (who suffered cognitive impairment).

So we know that berries have antioxidants and a powerful effect on the human brain to stave off memory loss in many instances. Your brain has to protect existing connections, but it also needs to heal any injuries at times.

Blueberries have been shown to protect the part of the brain that delivers access to your short-term memories. They also help with the creation of neurogenesis, which allows for the storage of new memories.

When you're planning your meals, you want to include foods that help the communication flow in your brain and maintain the number of healthy cells that you have to work with.

You want to adopt a diet that helps your entire body function at its best. You need plenty of blood flow and oxygen reaching your brain to keep things in tiptop shape.

We often hear people talk of a heart healthy diet, but you also want to make sure you're specifically adding brain healthy foods to your menu. Flavonoids (found in foods like kale and other leafy greens), help support your memory.

Other flavonoid foods you want to add to your diet are:

- Berries
- Apricots
- Pears
- Pinto and Black Beans
- Red Onions
- Apples
- Cabbage
- Tomatoes
- Parsley

Folate is a brain booster, too. You want to consume plenty of foods with folic acid with vitamin B12. That means, eating foods such as:

- Spinach
- Asparagus
- White Navy Beans
- Lentils

- Broccoli
- Cereal fortified with folic acid

Don't worry that it's too late to reverse signs of memory damage. Anytime you can help clean and repair nerves and cells by restoring them to good health, you can see signs of improvement!

Chapter 11: How to Control and Cure Cancer with Nutrition

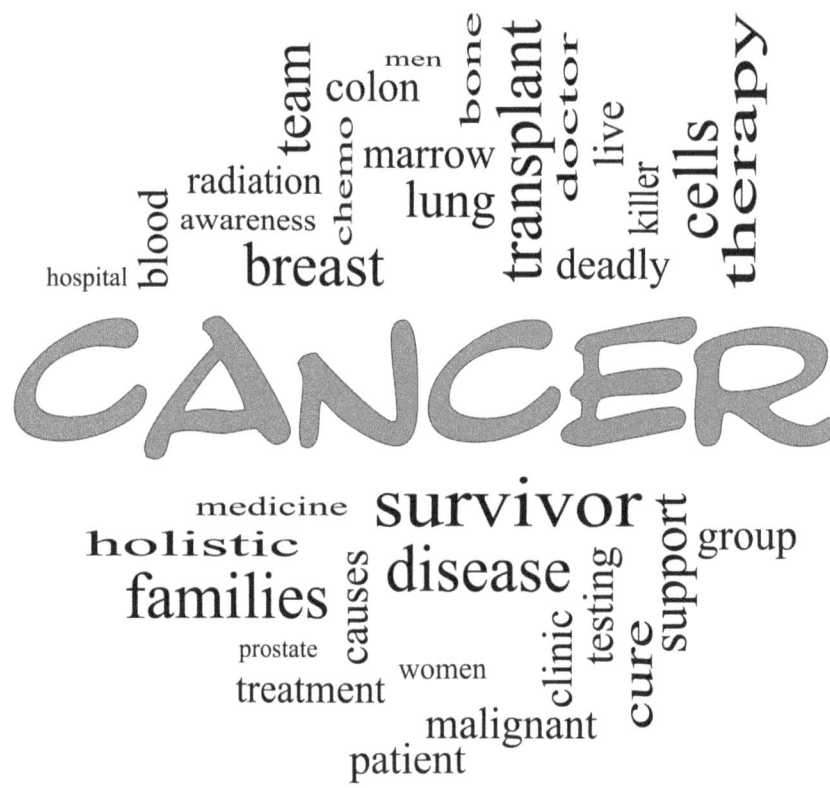

Cancer. It's one of the most feared words in our vocabulary and regardless of which type it is or how early it's detected, it strikes fear in our hearts. No one is fully immune to cancer – it can strike at any age in both genders.

Experts now know there are ways to reduce our risk. Part of that stems from early detection and vigilance in getting your screenings done on time. That's preventative and life-saving.

There may not be anything you can do about hereditary qualities, but they know that keeping a trim waistline and getting up and exercising is another way to keep cancer at bay.

Food is another thing you can control to manage your risk of developing cancer. Not only is it about the types of foods that you eat (or miss out on for protection), but it's about the way those foods are cooked.

Charcoal grills might make your food taste wonderful, but the cooking method of charring your food increases your body's risk for developing cancer – even when you thought grilling was naturally healthy!

It's the high temperatures that cause the most damage – so if you do grill your food, don't overcook it or char it to the point where it ignites the cancer causing chemicals to get released into your body.

Get Rid of Cancer Causing Toxins

Foods in slight moderation aren't going to harm your health to a strong degree. Enjoying the occasional treat is okay, but don't make these foods part of your regular diet – because that's when they become toxic.

Meats are generally cancer-causing foods – especially if they're processed like sandwich meat (bologna), hot dogs, sausage and more. Bacon is one of the worst offenders – and it's highly due to the sodium nitrate involved, along with all of the additives and preservatives.

When nitrates get into your body, they can be converted into nitrosamines. These cause cancer to develop and studies have shown that processed meat eaters are twice as likely to suffer from colorectal cancer, more likely to have stomach cancer and have an increased risk of getting pancreatic cancer, too.

Even if it's not processed, red meat can be a cancer trigger anyway. Beef consumption has been linked to the above cancers, as well as prostate, colon and breast cancer, too.

If you're trying to keep cancer at bay, meat isn't the only thing that you have to lay off. You also need to stay away from fried foods. Everything from potato chips and French fries to doughnuts help contribute to cancer in your body.

The snack foods often have carcinogens in them that are released again, during high temperatures. This is one reason why so many health advocates follow a mostly raw food diet – because cooking not only destroys nutrients, but it activates cancer causing elements.

It's not just potatoes that have this chemical – acrylamide - in them. Many foods that are heated to high degrees end up with this danger attached to them, but potatoes are the most susceptible to it.

Sugar doesn't just lead to obesity, which contributes to the development of cancer. Sugar is known to feed cancer cells, and it can speed up the development of cancer in your body.

You want to do everything you can to slow the process down. Cells in general are attracted to sugar – even the good cells in your body. But cancer cells take that sugar and use it to increase their power and destruction in your body.

Studies about sugar and the cancer connection have proven that men and women who consume more sugar and foods higher in the glycemic index are more likely to develop cancer.

What kinds of cancers do high sugar diets cause?

- Pancreatic
- Skin
- Uterine
- Urinary
- Breast

Next to heart disease, cancer is the second largest killer of men and women in the United States. So not only do you need to get rid of toxins, but you have to learn how to properly feed your body for protection, too.

Prevent the Growth of Cancer Cells By Eating These Foods

Recent studies show that diets high in animal protein are linked to an increased risk of cancer. But over age sixty-five, the rules change. If you eat meat, make sure it's grass-fed beef. That type of beef contains CLA, which stands for conjugated linoleic acid, which researchers feel helps fight cancer cell development.

To protect yourself from the development or growth of cancer cells, make sure you consume foods that empower your body at a cellular level. That means focusing on antioxidants.

These are foods that inhibit oxidation in your cells. This is what helps cancer cells generate and thrive inside your body, wreaking havoc on your healthy cells until you start showing signs and symptoms of disease.

Nuts are great for cancer protection. Peanuts and almonds have vitamin E, which help reduce the instances of cancer. Vitamin E supplements don't have the same effect on your body.

Your body needs fiber to function properly, so you want to eat plenty of whole grains (not white grains) that will help flush out toxins and keep your system clean.

Fruits, such as grapefruit, berries, and oranges provide antioxidant protection for your body. You want to choose foods rich in vitamin C, because that plays a role in keep cancer cell growth under control.

Berries in particular are known for their strong antioxidants – with blueberries ranking number one. Cranberries come in a close second. Both of these berries contain a high dose of cancer fighting antioxidants.

Vegetables that do the same include bell peppers and broccoli. Sweet potatoes pack a punch when it comes to fighting against cancer. The beta carotene in them is what helps so much.

Remember – supplements are not a good enough substitute for real, solid foods when it comes to giving your cells the nutrients they need to fight disease in your body.

Don't just rely on food alone in your fight to stay healthy against disease. In addition to solid foods, herbs and spices can also help keep you healthy. They can serve as anti-inflammatory agents and antioxidants, too.

Keeping your health intact is a burden that falls on your shoulders. Traditional medicine can only do so much to help you in the event disaster strikes. Ultimately, it's up to you to feed your body what it needs to survive – and protect it from toxic waste that prevents it from doing its job.

Meet the Author

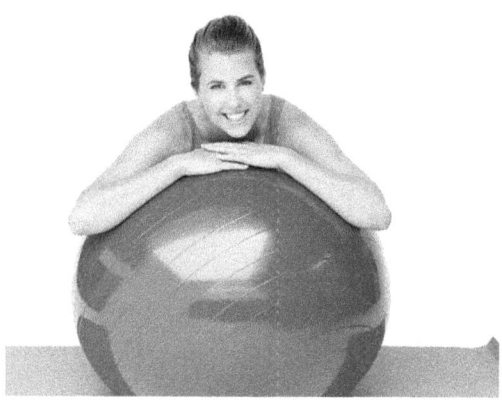

Certified personal trainer, nutrition and diet specialist and a wellness coach Kelly Larson's goal is to give as many people as possible the tools to start living a healthier lifestyle.

Kelly believes that every person can achieve the body of their dreams through fitness, healthy eating and a balanced lifestyle. Kelly follows her own personal health and fitness philosophies and believes that a "perfect body" is not a realistic goal. The importance of good health should drive and motivate people to achieve better fitness and a better body. When you take care of your body as a whole you will start to feel better and your body will transform into looking better.

Kelly lives in sunny Florida and enjoys spending time with family and friends. Kelly is passionate about music, scuba diving and new adventures. In her spare time, Kelly volunteers at her local animal shelter.

MORE BOOKS BY KELLY LARSON

Your Beach Body Transformation Begins Today: The Ultimate Guide to a Hot Summer Body

Six Pack Abs: How to Get Ripped Abs: The Truth on How to Reveal Your Six Pack Abs with Diet and Exercise

Green Tea for Weight Loss and Health: Detox, Boost Immunity, Lower Cholesterol, Increase Metabolism, Burn Calories and More

www.ingramcontent.com/pod-product-compliance
Ingram Content Group UK Ltd.
Pitfield, Milton Keynes, MK11 3LW, UK
UKHW051659240426
12048UKWH00039B/1516